FROM MANAGING TO CONQUERING ALDULT ACUTE MYELOID LEAKIA

Expert Guide To Understanding Adult Acute Myeloid Leakemia Causes, Symptoms, Preventing, Treatment For Optimal Wellness

DR. DASHIELL DANIEL

Disclaimer

This book, is intended to provide information and guidance on the subject matter and is not a substitute for professional medical advice, diagnosis, or treatment.

The author, is not a medical professional, and the content presented here is based on research, general knowledge, and expert guidance available at the time of writing.

The information in this book is provided with the understanding that the author and the publisher are not engaged in rendering medical, legal, or other professional services.

Any reliance on the information contained in this book is at the reader's own risk.

While every effort has been made to ensure the accuracy and completeness of the information presented, medical knowledge is constantly evolving, and new research may supersede the content in this book. The author and the publisher make no representations or warranties of any kind, express or implied, about the completeness, accuracy, reliability, suitability, or availability concerning the information, products, services, or related graphics contained in this book.

This book may contain references or mentions of individuals, products, websites, organizations, or other names for informational purposes only.

The author does not own or endorse any such entities mentioned in the book. Any resemblance to actual persons, living or dead, or actual events is purely coincidental.

Readers are encouraged to consult with qualified healthcare professionals for medical advice, diagnosis, and treatment tailored to their specific circumstances.

The author and the publisher disclaim any liability for any loss or risk, personal or otherwise, arising directly or indirectly from the use of the information presented in this book.

By reading this book, the reader acknowledges and agrees to the terms of this disclaimer.

In the fields of nematology and oncology, the book "Adult Acute Myeloid Leukemia" is extremely valuable as it provides a thorough examination of all the aspects related to this intricate hematologic cancer. This book's main goal is to provide a thorough understanding of adult acute myeloid leukemia (AML) to researchers, healthcare professionals, and students by acting as an authoritative reference. Hematologists, oncologists, nurses, medical students, and other allied health professionals involved in the treatment of AML patients are among the intended audience members.

The description, categorization, and pathophysiology of AML are explained in detail in the first few chapters, which lay a solid basis.

By exploring the complex terrain of AML subtypes, genetic variables, and risk factors, the book establishes the foundation for a comprehensive understanding of the illness.

In Chapter 1, clinically important insights are provided on the symptoms, indicators, and diagnostic techniques.

Using a statistical method, Chapter 2 deconstructs the epidemiology of AML, emphasizing its frequency, incidence, demographic trends, and worldwide effects. The risk factors and predisposing circumstances are covered in detail in later chapters, which are followed by a thorough examination of the AML diagnosis procedure and staging.

The book's core is found in Chapter 5, which carefully reviews the various AML therapy options. Every aspect is thoroughly examined, ranging from targeted medicines and supportive care to stem cell transplants and chemotherapy. In Chapter 6, we look ahead at AML therapy through the lens of emerging medicines and continuing research.

A distinctive aspect of the book may be discovered in Chapter 7, which discusses quality of life and survivability issues.

AML survivor psychosocial issues, long-term repercussions, and managing treatment side effects are covered in depth.

In conclusion, Chapter 8 brings a human element to the scholarly conversation by integrating the viewpoints of patients and caregivers.

A comprehensive understanding of the AML experience is provided via personal accounts, coping mechanisms, and readily available support services.

"Adult Acute Myeloid Leukemia" is essentially a valuable resource that bridges the gap between scientific understanding and real-world experience. It gives medical practitioners a thorough grasp of AML while acknowledging the complex difficulties that patients and their caregivers experience. With its substantial contribution to the field's collective knowledge and care methods, this book is expected to have a long-lasting influence on the landscape of AML literature.

Overview

Within the field of hematologic cancers, acute myeloid leukemia (AML) is a dangerous foe because of its unchecked growth of myeloid precursors in the bone marrow and peripheral circulation. Diagnostic, therapeutic, and management problems with this aggressive haematological illness are substantial.

This thorough investigation attempts to clarify the complex aspects of adult AML by exploring its molecular foundations, diagnostic approaches, treatment plans, and the constantly changing field of study.

The Book's Objective

This book's main goal is to function as an academic encyclopedia, clarifying the various facets of adult AML. It seeks to close the knowledge gap between clinical practice and the rapidly expanding body of information on the subject by offering a thorough resource to researchers, students, and healthcare professionals. Through the integration of the most recent scientific findings, clinical perspectives, and treatment innovations, the book aims to provide a comprehensive comprehension of AML.

The ultimate objectives are to equip physicians with evidence-based knowledge to improve patient treatment, encourage researchers to pursue new directions, and enlighten students on the complexities of this haematological cancer.

Intended Audience

This book has been carefully written to appeal to a wide range of readers, including researchers, students, and healthcare professionals. This database will be extremely helpful to hematologists, oncologists, pathologists, and other physicians who diagnose and treat hematologic malignancies. Hematology and oncology researchers will find a plethora of material to support their research and add to the growing body of knowledge. The organized insights into AML will also help medical students, residents, and fellows gain a better understanding of this complicated illness.

An Overview Of Acute Myeloid Leukemia (AML) In Adults

The clonal growth of myeloid precursors at the cost of normal hematopoiesis characterizes adult AML, which is used as a model for malignant transformation within the hematopoietic system. This cancerous condition results from genetic changes that provide hematopoietic stem and progenitor cells an advantage in proliferating.

The buildup of immature myeloid blasts in the peripheral blood and bone marrow, which causes cytopenias and raises the risk of bleeding and infections, is one of the characteristics of AML.

To provide a more accurate diagnosis and prognosis, the World Health Organization (WHO) classifies AML based on cytogenetic and molecular abnormalities.

AML diagnosis requires a careful fusion of genetic, morphological, immunophenotypic, and clinical evaluations. Flow cytometry, bone marrow aspirates, and peripheral blood smears are essential tools for determining the distinctive characteristics of AML. Numerous recurring mutations have been identified thanks to recent developments in genomic profiling, which have improved risk assessment and enabled more individualized treatment plans. A new era in the treatment of AML is being heralded by the development of targeted medicines and immunotherapeutic methods as our understanding of the disease's molecular landscape deepens.

We will cover AML etiology, clinical symptoms, diagnostic techniques, risk stratification, and changing therapy paradigms in this thorough investigation. To present a comprehensive view, the complex interactions among genetic abnormalities, the dynamic microenvironment of the bone marrow, and the immune system's function in AML will be examined. In addition, the book will examine novel treatment approaches, such as stem cell transplantation and developing immunotherapies, as well as the difficulties presented by relapsed or refractory AML.

It is critical to recognize the changing character of adult AML as we set off on our academic adventure through its environment. The intricacies of AML are still being uncovered by ongoing research projects, opening the door for innovative treatment approaches and diagnostic instruments. With its combination of present information and emerging viewpoints, this book seeks to be a guiding light in the constantly changing field of adult AML.

CHAPTER ONE
UNDERSTANDING ADULT ACUTE MYELOID LEUKEMIA

The haematological malignancy known as adult acute myeloid leukemia (AML) is typified by the fast growth of aberrant myeloid progenitor cells in the bone marrow and peripheral circulation. Sorting AML into several subtypes according to its morphological, cytogenetic, and molecular features occurs in the classification process.

The prognosis and treatment choices are greatly influenced by these subgroups. AML is also largely influenced by genetic variables; different subtypes and clinical outcomes are linked to certain mutations and chromosomal abnormalities.

The French-American-British (FAB) classification method, which takes into account the appearance of leukemia cells under a microscope, is used to categorize AML subtypes. This is further refined by the World Health Organization (WHO) categorization system, which incorporates molecular and genetic data. AML with recurring genetic abnormalities, AML with alterations due to myelodysplasia,

AML related to treatment, and AML not otherwise described are common subtypes. Distinctive features of every subtype impact its behavior, reaction to therapy, and general outlook.

The genetic components of AML are many and complex. Genes including FLT3, NPM1, CEBPA, and RUNX1 frequently exhibit mutations that impact prognosis. The heterogeneity of AML is influenced by chromosomal abnormalities, including deletions, inversions, and translocations affecting the MLL gene. Not only does the identification of these genetic variations facilitate the categorization of subtypes, but it also provides the basis for targeted therapy.

Age, exposure to specific environmental pollutants (like benzene), prior chemotherapy or radiation therapy, and specific genetic abnormalities (like Down syndrome) are among the risk factors linked to the development of AML. Knowing these risk factors is essential for identifying high-risk individuals and, where practical, putting preventative measures in place.

The typical process of blood cell growth and the pathophysiology of AML are closely related. Hematopoietic stem cells undergo progressive development into adult blood cells throughout the process of hematopoiesis in a healthy person.

This process is hampered in AML, which results in the build-up of immature myeloid cells. Leukemia cells infiltrate peripheral circulation and other organs, causing bone marrow failure due to unchecked growth and defective differentiation.

AML can appear in a variety of ways and is frequently vague. Symptoms that patients may encounter include weakness, weariness, fever, and easy bruising. Hepatomegaly and splenomegaly are two examples of organomegaly caused by leukemia cells invading different organs. Individual differences exist in the intensity and mix of symptoms, which are impacted by the leukemia's aggressiveness, age, and general health.

To establish the diagnosis of AML and identify its subtype, diagnostic techniques are essential. Abnormal numbers of white blood cells, red blood cells, and platelets are revealed by blood tests such as peripheral blood smears and complete blood counts (CBCs). To evaluate the cellular morphology, verify the existence of blast cells, and gather material for cytogenetic and molecular research, bone marrow aspiration and biopsy are necessary. Genetic tests and flow cytometry provide further support for subtype categorization and help direct treatment choices.

A thorough comprehension of adult acute myeloid leukemia includes knowledge of its description, categorization, risk factors, genetic makeup, and pathogenesis. The interaction of these variables affects the clinical presentation and prognosis of AML, adding to its variability. The development of individualized treatment techniques has been made possible by advancements in genetic and molecular profiling, which highlights the significance of precise subtype categorization for customized treatments. In the complicated world of AML, early detection with suitable diagnostic methods is still essential for starting prompt and efficient therapeutic measures.

CHAPTER TWO
STATISTICS AND EPIDEMIOLOGY

The hematological malignancy known as adult acute myeloid leukemia (AML) is typified by the fast growth of aberrant myeloid cells in the bone marrow and peripheral circulation. It is essential to comprehend the epidemiology and statistics of AML to guide clinical care, inform research activities, and evaluate the disease's impact on public health.

Incidence And Prevalence

The frequency and incidence of AML vary significantly throughout age groups and populations. AML is more common in elderly persons and has an increasing frequency as people age. Globally, the total prevalence varies, and there are geographical inequalities that may be related to environmental variables, healthcare facilities, and genetic predispositions.

It is difficult to estimate the incidence of AML accurately since diagnostic criteria and reporting methods differ. An increased risk factor is still advanced age, with a peak incidence seen in people over 65. Planning for healthcare and allocating resources requires an understanding of these prevalent trends, particularly for aging populations.

Patterns Of Demography

An important determinant in the incidence and prognosis of AML is demographics.

Gender disparities have been noted, with a somewhat greater frequency in men than in women. Variations in susceptibility and results can also be attributed to certain genetic and ethnic origins. For example, various ethnic groups may have varying frequencies of certain genetic variants linked to AML.

The socioeconomic determinants of AML demographics may also include healthcare availability. Examining these demographic subtleties is essential to better delivering healthcare services to a variety of communities and customizing preventative measures.

Rates Of Survivall

The aggressive nature of AML is well-known, and several variables, including patient age, genetic alterations, response to treatment, and general health state, might affect survival rates.

The prognosis for AML varies greatly, and older persons often have worse prognoses than younger ones. Recent years have seen improvements in survival rates due in part to developments in treatment techniques like as targeted medicines and stem cell transplantation. But problems still exist, and relapse is always a big worry.

Examining the variables influencing differences in survival rates yields important information for improving supporting care, adjusting treatment plans, and creating new therapeutic initiatives.

AML's Worldwide Effects

Beyond just hurting specific individuals, AML has an international influence on economies, societal well-being, and healthcare systems.

The burden of AML is high, and the expenses of diagnosis, treatment, and supportive care are high in the healthcare system. The interaction of genetic, environmental, and healthcare variables is reflected in the global distribution of AML patients. Regional differences in results are partly caused by differences in access to healthcare services. AML has an economic impact on missed productivity and caregiver expenses in addition to direct medical expenditures.

Advocating for enhanced healthcare infrastructure, allowing international research cooperation, and promoting fair access to effective therapies all depend on an understanding of the worldwide implications of anti-money laundering (AML).

Adult Acute Myeloid Leukemia epidemiology and statistics offer a thorough picture of the disease's frequency, demographic trends, survival rates, and worldwide effect. To effectively allocate resources, create targeted therapies, and address the complex issues surrounding AML globally, doctors, researchers, and governments must have this information.

CHAPTER THREE
PREDISPOSING CONDITIONS AND RISK FACTORS

A complicated hematologic malignancy, adult acute myeloid leukemia (AML) is defined by the fast growth of aberrant myeloid progenitor cells in the bone marrow and blood. AML is caused by a complex interaction of medical, environmental, and hereditary factors. It is essential to comprehend the risk factors and predisposing situations linked to AML to avoid and diagnose this aggressive illness early on.

The development of AML is significantly influenced by genetic factors. This kind of leukemia is predisposed in certain persons by inherited mutations in specific genes. The existence of certain chromosomal abnormalities, such as translocations involving chromosomes 15 and 17, which result in the creation of the PML-RARA fusion gene, is the most well-known genetic component linked to AML. In addition, AML sufferers commonly include mutations in genes such as FLT3, NPM1, and CEBPA. Finding these genetic markers helps with risk assessment as well as the creation of personalized targeted treatments based on a patient's genetic profile.

An important additional factor raising the chance of getting AML is the environment. There is evidence linking an increased prevalence of AML to exposure to certain carcinogens, including benzene and ionizing radiation.

Because of its leukemogenic qualities, benzene is a common industrial chemical that has been linked to an increased risk of developing AML in the workplace. Ionizing radiation can cause genetic alterations in hematopoietic cells, which can lead to leukemogenesis. This can occur from both medical therapies and occupational sources of radiation. For those who are vulnerable, avoiding AML requires an understanding of these environmental variables and reducing their exposure to them.

Prior medical treatments, including radiation and chemotherapy, are known risk factors for AML. Although these therapies are essential for treating different types of cancer, they may have long-term effects on the hematological system.

Secondary AML has been associated with specific chemotherapeutic drugs, including topoisomerase II inhibitors and alkylating agents.

AML is a dose-dependent late-stage consequence of cancer treatment that is more likely to occur in patients who have had numerous rounds of chemotherapy or radiation therapy. Oncology continues to face the difficult task of striking a careful balance between reducing the risk of subsequent AML and successfully treating the original tumor.

Additionally, predisposing medical factors may have a role in the development of AML. Immune system disorders such as aplastic anemia and myelodysplastic syndromes (MDS) make a person more susceptible to leukemic transformation.

With its inefficient haematopoiesis and cytopenias, MDS is a preleukemic disease that has the potential to develop into AML in the future. Comparably, leukemic clones can arise in an environment that is favorable to aplastic anemia, a disease marked by bone marrow failure.

It is crucial to comprehend the relationship between these underlying medical issues and the likelihood of AML in identifying high-risk patients and putting effective monitoring plans in place.

Adult acute myeloid leukemia is connected with a variety of complex risk factors and predisposing diseases. Particular chromosomal abnormalities and mutations in important genes are examples of genetic variables that greatly contribute to individual vulnerability. The risk is further increased by environmental variables, such as exposure to ionizing radiation and toxins like benzene.

A dose-dependent incidence of secondary AML is associated with prior medical therapies, particularly radiation therapy and chemotherapy, underscoring the need for meticulous treatment planning. Health problems that predispose people to developing AML include aplastic anemia and multiple developmental disorders (MDS).

To manage adult acute myeloid leukemia, a thorough understanding of these characteristics is essential for risk assessment, prevention, and the development of focused therapy methods.

CHAPTER FOUR
DIAGNOSIS AND STAGING

The hematologic malignancy known as adult acute myeloid leukemia (AML) is typified by the fast growth of aberrant myeloid cells in the bone marrow, which impairs the synthesis of healthy blood cells. Using a variety of diagnostic techniques, a thorough examination is necessary for the diagnosis and staging of AML.

The main ideas of diagnosis and staging, including blood tests, bone marrow aspiration and biopsy, imaging examinations, and AML staging systems, will be covered in detail in this part.

Blood tests are essential for the preliminary assessment of AML because they offer vital information about hematologic parameters. Abnormalities in the counts of white blood cells, red blood cells, and platelets can be found with the use of a Complete Blood Count (CBC) with differential.

Leucocytosis, anemia, and thrombocytopenia are the most common symptoms of AML. Additionally, blast cells—immature cells characteristic of leukemia—may be seen in peripheral blood smears. Characterizing the immunophenotype of leukemic cells by flow cytometry helps to classify them into subtypes and informs treatment choices.

AML diagnostic confirmation and vital information on the degree of disease involvement are achieved through the use of bone marrow aspiration and biopsy. A biopsy includes taking out a tiny core of bone and marrow tissue, whereas aspiration involves taking out a liquid sample from the marrow. After that, a microscope examination of these samples allows for the evaluation of genetic anomalies, immunophenotypes, and cell morphology. AML is characterized by a large number of blast cells in the bone marrow, which helps with diagnosis and prognostic categorization.

Assessing the degree of AML and identifying extramedullary involvement are aided by imaging tests. Imaging modalities including magnetic resonance imaging (MRI) and computed tomography (CT) scans can detect organ infiltration by leukemic cells, which helps with treatment planning even though they are not usually utilized for initial diagnosis. When assessing lymph node enlargement, liver and spleen involvement, and the existence of chloromas (extramedullary masses of leukemic cells), these investigations are very helpful.

To assess risk and direct therapy choices for AML patients, staging systems are essential instruments. The French-American-British (FAB) classification is the most often used staging method. It divides AML into subtypes according to the morphological and cytochemical properties of the blast cells. The World Health Organization (WHO) classification is another significant classification system that uses molecular genetic and cytogenetic data to identify AML subtypes. The prognostic importance of molecular markers including FLT3, NPM1, and CEBPA mutations is becoming more well-acknowledged.

A crucial component of AML staging is cytogenetic analysis, which pinpoints certain chromosomal abnormalities with predictive value.

For example, positive outcomes are linked to the existence of t(8;21), inv(16), or t(15;17) translocations, but complicated karyotypes or particular anomalies such as monosomy 5 or 7 are suggestive of a bad prognosis. The selection of suitable treatment options, such as the investigation of hematopoietic stem cell transplantation in high-risk situations, is guided by these cytogenetic results.

Adult acute myeloid leukemia is diagnosed and staged using a multimodal method that includes imaging scans, blood testing, bone marrow aspiration and biopsy, and extensive staging systems. When combined, these techniques help control AML by providing precise diagnosis, risk assessment, and well-informed treatment choices. Our understanding of AML heterogeneity has improved with the integration of cytogenetic and molecular data, opening the door to individualized therapy approaches catered to the unique genetic profile of each patient. The field's ongoing research is improving diagnostic and staging paradigms, which gives promise for better results in the difficult AML management environment.

CHAPTER FIVE
METHODS OF TREATMENT

AML, or adult acute myeloid leukemia, is a complicated and aggressive hematologic cancer that spreads quickly across the bone marrow and peripheral circulation. To obtain the best results, managing AML requires a multifaceted strategy that combines several treatment approaches. Chemotherapy is a key component of the treatment toolbox for AML.

The mainstay of AML treatment is chemotherapy, which tries to kill leukemia cells to bring about remission. Strong cytotoxic drugs like cytarabine and anthracyclines are given as part of induction treatment, the first stage of chemotherapy.

The goal of this rigorous therapy is to lower the leukemia load to an undetectable level so that normal hematopoiesis can return. Since induction therapy lays the groundwork for later treatments, it is essential to the overall outcome of treatment.

Consolidation therapy is, therefore, necessary to remove any remaining leukemia cells and stop the illness from relapsing after induction therapy. Additional chemotherapy cycles are usually administered as part of consolidation therapy, frequently with new drugs or at greater dosages. Eliminating any leukemic cells that may still be present will increase the likelihood of a long-lasting remission. A personalized consolidation regimen is chosen after taking into account the patient's age, cytogenetics, and induction treatment response.

While it's not always used, maintenance treatment could be taken into consideration in some situations to extend remission and lower the chance of recurrence. Maintenance usually entails longer-term, reduced dosages of targeted medicines or chemotherapy. Maintenance therapy tries to further inhibit any remaining leukemia cells that may not have been destroyed during previous treatment phases. It is carefully chosen to balance efficacy and potential long-term negative effects.

Stem cell transplantation becomes an important therapeutic alternative, particularly when chemotherapy isn't working to cure a patient's condition. The process of autologous transplantation entails reconstituting the bone marrow with the patient's hematopoietic stem cells, which are harvested and kept throughout remission. On the other side, allogeneic transplantation makes use of stem cells from a compatible donor, frequently a matched sibling or unrelated person. The use of allogeneic approaches carries the risk of graft-versus leukemia effects, in which immune cells from donors target leukemia cells that are still present, adding another degree of anti-leukemic activity.

The treatment of AML has undergone a radical change with the introduction of targeted treatments. These treatments allow for more targeted and less harmful interventions by concentrating on particular genetic or cellular defects in leukemia cells. Tyrosine kinase inhibitors, like gilteritinib and midostaurin, for instance, target specific mutations like FLT3, improving outcomes for patients with AML that have this mutation. As our knowledge of AML biology expands, so does the way targeted therapies are incorporated into treatment algorithms.

To address the various problems and difficulties related to AML and its treatment, supportive care is essential to the overall management of the illness. An essential component of supportive care, blood transfusions aid in the management of anemia and thrombocytopenia brought on by the illness and its treatment. Infections are a major source of morbidity and death in patients with AML, and antibiotic medication is essential for controlling and avoiding them, especially when chemotherapy-induced immunosuppression is in effect. To minimize the negative effects of chemotherapy and guarantee patient comfort and adherence to treatment regimens, antiemetic medication is crucial.

A complex and multifaceted strategy is used to treat adult acute myeloid leukemia, including supportive care, targeted treatments, chemotherapy, and stem cell transplantation.

The exact combination and order of these modalities are determined by the unique features of each patient, the biology of the disease, and the patient's reaction to early therapies.

Progress in the study of AML and ongoing research indicates that treatment approaches will be improved in the long run, benefiting those who are afflicted with this difficult hematologic cancer.

CHAPTER SIX
NEW THERAPIES AND RESEARCH

With the advent of innovative therapeutic techniques, the field of AML therapy has undergone a paradigm change in recent years. Immunotherapy is among the most promising approaches (6.1). Through immunotherapy, cancer cells are identified and eradicated by the body's immune system. AML patients may benefit greatly from several immunotherapy techniques, including chimeric antigen receptor (CAR) T-cell treatment and immune checkpoint inhibitors. Clinical studies are being conducted to investigate checkpoint inhibitors, which obstruct the inhibitory signals that cancer cells use to elude the immune system. Contrarily, CAR-T cells entail genetically altering a patient's T cells to express receptors that target AML cells, and they have shown promising outcomes in certain instances. More individualized and focused treatment approaches are made possible by the complex interactions between AML cells and the immune system.

Another area of focus in AML research is Novel Targeted Agents (6.2). Conventional chemotherapy frequently damages healthy cells inadvertently because it lacks selectivity.

On the other hand, targeted medicines seek to specifically interfere with pathways essential to the survival of cancer cells. It is being developed to target particularly the dysregulated proteins or mutations in AML cells with monoclonal antibodies and small compounds. For example, subgroups of AML patients have demonstrated the effectiveness of inhibitors of certain signaling pathways, such as FLT3 and IDH inhibitors. New targets are being found as a result of our growing understanding of the genetic and molecular heterogeneity of AML. This progress makes it possible to create therapeutic approaches that are less harmful and more targeted.

Clinical trials (6.3) are essential to the advancement of AML therapy. Because AML is so complicated and heterogeneous, new treatments must be rigorously tested across a range of patient groups. A large number of clinical trials are being conducted to assess the effectiveness and safety of new medicines. Phase II and III studies examine the novel treatment's efficacy in greater detail and contrast it with conventional methods, whereas Phase I trials concentrate on the safety profile, dose, and any adverse effects. To plan and carry out these studies, cooperation between academic institutions, pharmaceutical corporations, and regulatory agencies is essential. The continual development of AML therapies is facilitated by the ongoing improvement of trial designs, the integration of biomarker-driven strategies, and the investigation of novel outcomes.

Further advancements in patient outcomes are possible, as shown by Future Directions in AML Treatment (6.4). It is anticipated that the incorporation of genetic and molecular profiling into standard clinical practice would improve the ability to identify certain mutations and changes, enabling the development of more individualized treatment plans. With its focus on customized treatment regimens based on genetic profiles, precision medicine is probably going to become more widespread. Furthermore, there is now research being done on the evaluation of combination treatments, which include a careful mixture of conventional chemotherapy, targeted medicines, and immunotherapy. Interventions that target the leukemic cells' supporting habitat may present new opportunities for therapeutic development as our understanding of the AML microenvironment expands. Moreover, given the special difficulties that older individuals present in terms of treatment tolerance and comorbidities—a substantial fraction of AML cases—it is imperative that efforts be made to develop medicines for these people.

The field of AML therapy is changing as a result of continuous study and development. Clinical trials, immunotherapy, and targeted agents are at the forefront of these developments. Prospects in AML therapy emphasize the significance of combination medicines, customized medicine, and a thorough knowledge of the biology behind the illness.

To convert these developments into significant therapeutic improvements for patients with adult acute myeloid leukemia, collaboration between researchers, doctors, and industry partners is essential.

CHAPTER SEVEN
SURVIVAL AND LIFE QUALITY

A vital component of adult Acute Myeloid Leukemia (AML) patients' journey past the acute stage of the disease is their quality of life and survival. This stage entails several difficulties, from treating the long-term impacts of AML therapy to controlling medication side effects.

Moreover, survivorship's psychological and emotional dimensions are crucial, necessitating all-encompassing care and support approaches. This is where the need to provide supportive care for survivors enters the picture, guaranteeing a comprehensive strategy to improve the general health of those who have overcome AML.

In AML, controlling treatment side effects is an essential part of survivorship care. Strong chemotherapy is a common part of AML treatment, and this can have a wide range of negative effects, from exhaustion and nausea to more serious issues including bleeding and infections.

A multidisciplinary strategy comprising oncologists as well as supportive care experts like nurses, dietitians, and pharmacists is needed to address these side effects. Prophylactic antibiotics to avoid infections, blood transfusions to address anemia, and antiemetic drugs to treat nausea are examples of management options. The goal is to improve the patient's entire quality of life both during and after therapy, in addition to ensuring that the treatment is effective.

The long-term effects of AML treatment complicate survivability even more. Following therapy, AML survivors may experience persistent health problems such as heart problems, follow-up malignancies, and infertility problems.

Some chemotherapeutic drugs have cardiotoxic effects that might lead to cardiovascular problems.

For AML survivors, maintaining and monitoring cardiovascular health becomes crucial in the long-term care strategy.

Furthermore, even with the minimal incidence of subsequent malignancies, close monitoring is necessary. Given the possible effects of AML therapy on reproductive health, fertility preservation techniques ought to be considered and put into practice as early in the therapeutic process as possible.

It is impossible to overestimate the psychological and emotional aspects of AML survival. AML patients frequently experience severe psychological suffering both during and after therapy. Common emotional issues include post-traumatic stress disorder, anxiety, sadness, and dread of recurrence. It is essential to incorporate mental health assistance into survival treatment. To address these emotional components, psychosocial therapies, counseling, and support groups are essential. Healthcare professionals must be sensitive to the mental health needs of AML survivors and work to create a culture that values and de-stigmatizes candid conversations regarding mental health.

Providing a wide range of therapies targeted at enhancing the general well-being of AML survivors is known as "Supportive Care for Survivors."

This entails controlling not just one's physical health but also one's social, spiritual, and financial facets of life following anti-money laundering. Plans for survivorship care should incorporate health monitoring, instructional materials, and routine follow-up visits. Social support, such as participation in survivorship groups, facilitates connections between people who have experienced comparable difficulties and promotes a feeling of community.

A component of comprehensive supportive care includes also addressing existential and spiritual issues. In addition, given the potential financial strain that cancer treatment may have on survivors, financial advice and support are essential.

In adult acute myeloid leukemia, survival extends beyond the end of active therapy. It entails a thorough strategy for handling side effects of therapy, dealing with long-term impacts, promoting mental and emotional health, and offering general supportive care. Healthcare providers may make a substantial contribution to improving the quality of life for those who have overcome hematologic malignancy by identifying and attending to the unique requirements of AML survivors.

CHAPTER EIGHT
VIEWS OF THE PATIENT AND THE CAREGIVER

The diagnosis of acute myeloid leukemia (AML) is difficult and complex, and it has a significant effect on patients as well as those who care for them. Physical and psychological hardships are common during the AML journey, therefore a thorough knowledge of both the patient's and the caregiver's perspectives is necessary to improve holistic treatment.

Individual Narratives

Personal narratives are essential for clarifying the complex realities of those dealing with AML.

These narratives offer a personal description of the emotional rollercoaster that followed the diagnostic journey and various therapeutic options. Patients describe their physical symptoms, uncertainty about the diagnosis, and the psychological effects of dealing with a life-threatening illness. Not only do personal narratives illuminate the many forms of AML, but they also provide motivation and fortitude to those encountering comparable difficulties.

Adaptive Techniques

Managing an AML diagnosis calls for a multimodal strategy that takes into account practical, psychological, and emotional factors.

To manage the uncertainty around their therapy, side effects, and general quality of life, patients frequently utilize coping mechanisms.

Creating a support system, practicing mindfulness, and getting professional psychiatric help are a few examples of these tactics. The comprehension and application of efficacious coping strategies are crucial elements in alleviating the psychological strain linked to AML, thereby enhancing the general welfare of both those receiving care and those providing it.

Resources and Support Groups

Resources and support groups are essential for building a feeling of community and offering priceless aid to those impacted by AML.

These organizations allow patients and caregivers a forum to talk about their experiences, share information, and get emotional support from people who understand the particular difficulties presented by AML. Additionally, having access to instructional materials gives patients and caregivers the information they need to decide on long-term care, possible side effects, and treatment alternatives. Building and maintaining a support system may greatly improve the coping strategies of those impacted by AML, making the community more resilient and knowledgeable. later

It is critical to provide patient-centered care by understanding the viewpoints of both the patient and the caregiver in the setting of adult acute myeloid leukemia.

Personal narratives illuminate both the challenges and the successes of the individual journey through AML, offering a deeper view of the experience. Coping mechanisms are crucial instruments for managing the intricacies of the diagnosis, which comprise mental, emotional, and functional aspects. Resources and support groups are essential cornerstones that provide knowledge essential for making well-informed decisions and cultivating a feeling of community. By incorporating these ideas into clinical practice, AML treatment may be provided in a comprehensive manner that addresses the psychological factors that have a significant impact on patients' and caregivers' well-being in addition to the medical ones.

CONCLUSION

The complicated biology and inconsistent response to therapy of Acute Myeloid Leukemia (AML), a heterogeneous hematological malignancy, provide a considerable therapeutic challenge. More accurate diagnoses and focused treatments have been made possible in recent years by growing knowledge of the disease's molecular and genetic landscape. This thorough examination of AML covers important ideas about the disease's biology, diagnostics, treatment options, and the changing field of clinical trials and research.

The disruption of normal hematopoiesis by genetic and molecular abnormalities is closely associated with the etiology of AML. Particularly important roles in leukemogenesis are played by mutations in genes including FLT3, NPM1, and CEBPA.

The unchecked growth and compromised differentiation of myeloid cells are further exacerbated by the deregulation of transcription factors and signaling pathways. Comprehending these molecular deviations not only improves the categorization of AML but also has potential applications in the creation of tailored treatments. New therapeutic targets are continually being discovered as scientists dive further into the complex biological processes, providing promise for more individualized and successful treatment plans.

A multidisciplinary approach that includes clinical, morphological, immunophenotypic, and molecular evaluations is used to diagnose AML.

Decisions about therapy are influenced by the detection of certain cytogenetic and molecular abnormalities, which also help with risk classification.

The development of next-generation sequencing has transformed AML molecular profiling and made it possible to comprehend its heterogeneity on a much larger scale. The selection of customized treatment interventions is made easier and prognostication is improved when these diagnostic tools are included in ordinary clinical practice.

Over time, AML treatment approaches have changed dramatically, moving from conventional chemotherapy regimens to more sophisticated approaches that include hematopoietic stem cell transplantation (HSCT) and targeted treatments. Although cytarabine and anthracycline remain the cornerstone of treatment, the use of targeted medicines such as tyrosine kinase inhibitors has demonstrated encouraging outcomes, especially in individuals with certain genetic abnormalities. Individualized treatment planning and risk assessment are crucial, as allogeneic hematopoietic stem cell therapy (allogeneic HSCT) is a potentially curative alternative that is frequently investigated for suitable individuals.

Even with these developments, limiting treatment-related toxicities and attaining long-lasting remissions continue to present difficulties.

The fine-tuning of treatment strategies continues to revolve around striking the right balance between eliminating leukemic cells and maintaining normal hematopoiesis.

Immunotherapeutic approaches that use the immune system to specifically target leukemia cells, such as immune checkpoint inhibitors and chimeric antigen receptor T-cell treatment, are starting to show promise as game-changers.

AML research is a dynamic field with continuous efforts to understand the disease's intricacies and find new treatment approaches.

Accelerating the translation of scientific findings into clinical practice is the goal of collaborative projects like large-scale genome investigations and multinational clinical trials. A paradigm change towards precision medicine in AML may be facilitated by the incorporation of artificial intelligence and machine learning into data analysis, which might lead to more precise prognostication and treatment response prediction.

Acute myeloid leukemia in adults is a complex clinical entity influenced by complex molecular and genetic environments.

AML management is changing as a result of improvements in our knowledge of AML etiology, improved diagnostic techniques, and the developing of treatment plans. AML patients have a bright future thanks to the combination of immunotherapeutic modalities, targeted medicines, and ongoing research into the molecular details of the illness. The path towards more individualized, efficient, and minimally toxic therapeutic approaches for AML patients is approaching as long as research projects and clinical trials go on uncovering the intricacies of the disease.

www.ingramcontent.com/pod-product-compliance
Lightning Source LLC
Chambersburg PA
CBHW071128260726
48661CB00006B/2731